Here's an educational workbook for you:

„Your Guide to Positive Life
Volume II: Don't lose your energy!"

This is the second instalment in the series of original exercises which will help you learn how to use your life energy in a positive way.

As we work through it, you will be able to:
- Wake up full of positive energy, which will let you keep a good mood and motivation throughout the day;
- Plan your day to reduce day-to-day stress from unfinished matters you have been putting off;
- Open your heart to forgiveness and leave behind years' worth of hidden resentments;
- Ensure adequate rest and sleep;
- Develop assertiveness;
- Find the meaning of your life by accepting who you are and what you have;
- Restore your energy when you are surrounded by despair and doubt.

What if I told you that you can work on yourself and become someone you've always wanted to be? How would you feel about it?

You will find out for yourself that you can develop good habits thanks to the small changes described in this booklet!

This is your time. Take control of your
Life – Health – Relationships – Dreams

Remember! You're doing it all for yourself.

I wish you luck in discovering yourself!
Kasia Dorosz

Table of contents

How to work with *The Guid*? 3
Your daily plan 4
    Morning routine 4
    Evening routine 4
    Weekly tasks 5
1. Energy and stress 7
2. Positive attitude 9
3. Step-by-step planning 11
4. Your motivation 15
5. Acceptance 17
6. Declutter your surroundings 19
7. Sleep and rest 21
8. Assertiveness 23
9. Healthy eating and exercising 27
10. Anger and jealousy 31
11. Toxic people 35
12. Self care 37
Motivational sentences for you 39

Copyright © 2019 Katarzyna Dorosz

No part of this publication may be reproduced, stored in a retrieval system, or transmitted in any form or by any means, electronic, mechanical, photocopied, recorded, scanned without the prior written permission of the author.

How to work with The Guide

If you diligently worked through volume I of the Guide, you can proceed easily to the „Weekly Tasks" section and begin your journey towards a life full of energy.

If you haven't had the opportunity to read volume I, I encourage you to purchase it in the form of an ebook (pdf) to print from my website (acti50.TV). It is a detailed introduction to a whole series of Guides, currently in preparation. You will also find there a step-by-step discussion of the Plan of the Day, presented on the following pages of the present booklet.

To work with the Guide, you will need:

1. A book of inspiring sentences/scripture/other valuable read
Every morning, you will feed your mind and heart with inspiring content.

2. A notebook
Write down the answers to all the questions and exercises suggested in the Guide. It is very important to do it manually! This way you will be able to focus more on the answers and always be able to go back to them. You will see the results of your work from week to week. You can continue to write in the notebook from Volume I.

3. A book calendar
Use it every evening. It is your intimate place to write down notes and describe your experiences from the exercises you complete along the way.

Go back to them once a week to see how much progress you have made!

Remember, your thoughts are worth writing down!

Your daily plan

The morning and evening exercises presented below are a nice everyday routine we have developed while working on volume I of the Guide. This is what **ensures a balance between body and spirit.**

Morning routine

1. Gratitude practice

Strive to feel gratitude immediately after waking up. Finish the sentence: „I am grateful for..." or just say „Thank you". Focusing on the good that surrounds you will help you to start your day with joy.

2. An inspirational sentence

Read one sentence and contemplate it in silence. Focus on what value it brings to your life. Feed your heart!

3. Contemplation

Find a comfortable position for you to contemplate in. Focus on your breath and your heartbeat. Feel your whole body. Stay silent for 10 - 20 minutes.

4. Exercises for a good day

Do your favorite physical exercises. Let your body know that a new day has begun. You need its strength!

5. Affirmations

Repeat positive statements about yourself. For example, mine are as follows: "I am clever! I am respectable! I am a valuable person! I deserve all the best!

Evening routine

1. Relaxation.

It's time to spare a moment to take care of your body. Do a few short relaxing exercises to get rid of the tensions that may have accumulated during the day.

2. **Contemplation.**
   Find a comfortable position to contemplate in. Quiet your thoughts. Focus on your breath. Let everything that happened throughout the day out of your mind.

3. **Filling the calendar.**
   Answer the questions: What am I thankful for today? What good have I done today? What have I learned today? Write down one positive thought that crossed your mind today.

4. **Gratitude and good sleep**
   Frame the day with gratitude – be thankful for what happened to you today. Now go to bed feeling calm and free from your worries and with great trust and love for yourself and the world. Sleep well.

Weekly tasks

Every week we will discuss three topics. Set a time during the day when you will be able to focus on the materials in peace and quiet. Work on them conscientiously, one by one!

Week I	Energy and stress	Positive attitude	Step-by-step planning
Week II	Your motivation	Acceptance	Declutter your surroundings
Week III	Sleep and rest	Assertiveness	Healthy eating and exercising
Week IV	Anger and jealousy	Toxic people	Self care

Your Guide to Positive Life

1. ENERGY AND STRESS

What is the energy we have inside?
If we are to work on preserving energy, let us first determine what it actually is. **Energy is life.** An optimal level of energy in the physical, mental, and emotional sphere gives us a sense of well-being. As we age, various dysfunctions take away our life energy. Therefore, we should manage it well and learn how to replenish it. Step by step, I will show you how to do this.

How does stress affect our energy?
*Stress is not what happens to people,
it is how they react internally to particular situations.*

If the negative reaction to a situation lasts for a long time and is excessively intense, not only does it have a devastating effect on our bodies, but also creates a lot of nervous tension. Stress can burn out your energy in an instant. However, I have a few ways for you to help you restore the right mental balance:

- **Breathe**
It is worth learning to breathe deeply and in the right way, as it allows us to calm our thoughts and soothe our nerves.

- **Be active**
Just 30 minutes a day spent on a walk or morning gymnastics will reduce the level of cortisol, known as the stress hormone. Remember, regularity is important.

- **Spend time with your friends**
Relax, talk about your problems and look for ways to solve them together.

Exercise:
Make a list of all the things that make you excessively stressed. Take the time to look for solutions to these problems. Write down all the ideas, even the unrealistic ones. The next day, review the list again and see what you can actually do. Ask your loved ones for support. Put things you can't influence into God's care. Finally, go for a long, relaxing walk.

Your Guide to Positive Life

2. POSITIVE ATTITUDE

Now you know how to deal with the most stressful situations you've been involved in. **But how do you prevent new ones?** When you create dark scenarios and worry about the future, you suck the energy out of yourself. Continuous complaining has a negative effect on your well-being and health, it takes away the joy from your everyday life and the strength you need to keep going. It's time to end this spiral of dark thoughts and worries!

Make sure to maintain healthy optimism and mental hygiene – this will give you the right amount of energy. As a result, you will continue to enjoy life even in difficult situations you can't control.

Exercise:
1. Write down three affirmations that help you think positively about life. Add them to the list of affirmations you repeat every morning. These sentences help me to maintain the joy of lif
   - I deserve all the best.
   - I am my own best friend.
   - I am healthy, happy and have a positive attitude – this is what I'm like.
2. Write down three passions that you would like to pursue in your life.

Remember!
It is never too late to find your own interests. Take me as an example: I am 50 years old and I want to cultivate my love of dancing, travelling and inspiring people like you with my healthy lifestyle and serenity.

3. Write down your memory of the last time you learned something new because you wanted it. What was it? How did you feel?

Can you already see the connection between a positive attitude to life, developing your passions and gaining knowledge? All the activities we take up out of our own volition **give us the joy of life, increase our self-esteem and provide a wonderful boost of positive energy.**

Your Guide to Positive Life

3. STEP-BY-STEP PLANNING

Our last exercise has brought you to the point where you think: „I want to act! I want to live!". That's great. **You're most likely looking for the time to develop your passions.** Good planning will help you do that. You will be able to do exactly what you need to do to maintain the right levels of energy.

I recommend daily, weekly, monthly, quarterly and annual planning. Right now we are going to discuss the first three ways of planning and put them into practice. We will come back to quarterly and annual planning in the next Guides. **For now, I want you to feel confident in planning your everyday life – this is the first step to make change.**

Daily planning
Every evening, make a plan for the next day.

What time are you going to you get up? When are you going to spend time on the Morning, Evening, and Weekly Rituals? Plan time for your favorite physical activity and prepare a healthy and tasty meal.

Now write down **your remaining tasks for the next day** – you can order them by completion time or priority (the most important ones at the top of the list).

Keep your calendar open and visible so you can check it throughout he day keep truck of what's most important to you and gradually cross out what you've already done.

Remember!
You don't have to plan every minute of your life. Planning is all about finding time for things that are important to you. Focus on them. If you haven't finished something on a given day, move it to the next day in your calendar.

Weekly planning

On Sunday evening, take time to see the whole next week from a bird's-eye view. **Write down all the events that will take place in the coming days:** a meeting at a club, a doctor's appointment, a meeting with relatives. **Think about which days you would like to devote to developing your passions.** If, for example, you are a gardener, check the weather forecast to plan your work on warm and sunny days. If, on the other hand, you love to read books, see if it is not time to go to a library or bookstore for a new book..

Monthly planning

In the case of monthly planning, I encourage you to hang a calendar in a visible place on the wall, one with **separate pages for each month and a place for short notes.**

This calendar will serve as a guide to the most important events. Write down the most important things in real time: <u>time, date, venue and subject</u>. Note your regular activities here as well – if you go to regular meetings or group classes – write them down.

Thanks to this, when you make an appointment with friends, for example, you can see all your already set up meetings and activities in one place.

Exercise:

1. Plan your upcoming day, week and month. Now you know how!
2. Plan what you want to do in the next month for yourself, your family and your home. Write everything down on a separate list and include it in your monthly, weekly and daily schedule.

When you stick to your plan, you'll see how pleasant it is. You will feel organized externally and internally. This will have an impact on your entire life – better well-being, contact with loved ones, and an unexpected flow of energy. **Now you can feel that you have control over your life, which happens here and now.**

Workbook 2

Your Guide to Positive Life

4. YOUR MOTIVATION

What motivates me to plan and take care of my body and mind is the joy that comes with every well experienced day. The truth is that like everyone else, I am discouraged, tired and worried: „What is all this for? What is the meaning in this?" **When I feel a drop in energy, I know it's time to work on my motivation.** It is thanks to this that I still feel full of life.

Test my proven motivational methods:

1. **Fill your home with music**

   Choose the music you like. Make it energetic and full of happy sounds. Knowingly choose music that you can't ignore. Start humming or rocking to the rhythm a little bit. Don't feel embarrased.

2. **Befriend laughter therapy**

   Did you know that your brain can't tell the difference between real and fake laughter? Take advantage of it! Stand in front of a mirror and smile at yourself. You can also make a short „ha ha ha ha" with every breath until the laughter flows on its own. Does this seem difficult to you? Practice makes perfect, and laughing will relieve all the tension in your body, and the joy you feel will motivate you to act.

Now that you feel relaxed in your body and light in your spirit, take a look at your exercise book and calendar. See what goals you have decided to achieve and why. Imagine how you are going to feel when you achieve what is important to you.

Remember the exercise in the first volume of the Guide when you wrote down the small successes of the whole week? Let them be your encouragement to experience the upcoming good days.

Write down in your calendar how you felt today when you were working on your motivation.

Your Guide to Positive Life

5. ACCEPTANCE

"Do what you can, with what you have, where you are."
                                                    Roosvelt

We cannot control everything, and such things must be accepted. Tilting at windmills is a waste of energy which you can use to improve your life.

Accept life as it is and enjoy the place where you are. If there is something you cannot tolerate, see if you can change it.

Believe in yourself and find your own rhythm.

Exercises:

1. Create a list in the exercise book.
   Write down all the things you find hard to accept. Make sure that these are the type of things that touch your everyday life. Maybe you are sick and every day is marked by another dose of medicine? Maybe you are feeling lonely?

2. "Do what you can with what you have".
   Write down everything you can think of to help you change your situation.

3. "Do what you can (...) where you are".
   Think and write about how you can make better use of the place you live in? See the example below:

My situation	What can I do?
I live alone and have no close friends.	Love myrself and like my own company (acceptance). Get to know my neighbours. Check if there are any clubs or UTAs in my city. Go to the library or park and talk to the people I meet.

Your Guide to Positive Life

6. DECLUTTER YOUR SURROUNDINGS

Cyclical decluttering of your surroundings, but also your inner life, is another very important element thanks to which you will make room for new energy. By clearing your space, you will stop wasting your energy on cleaning up unnecessary objects! Your home will be clean and spacious for longer.

Declutter your surroundings at least once a year. Clean room after room, get rid of things that are damaged, useless and sucking energy out of you.

For example, start with clothes. Collect all your clothes in one place. Arrange them by category: underwear, trousers, sweaters, jackets, etc., and look at them one by one. Put back in the wardrobe only those that are comfortable and feel good. If the other things are in good condition, you can put them in containers for used clothes – let them be useful to others.

Remember!
Even if you stay at home be a well-groomed and tidy person. Stop wearing stretched and faded clothes. Dress comfortably but neatly. Do it for yourself.

Exercise:
1. Bring a new order to a new beginning!
   Following the above advice, add the time to clean the whole house to your monthly plan. Take a break between cleaning days to help you maintain your energy and avoid feeling overwhelmed. Half an hour a day is a lot!

2. Make a list of things you don't need, but it's hard to throw them away.
   Look for people who could enjoy your things. Ask your friends. You can also ask for help in selling them on Internet. For example, you can gift excess books to a library or a second-hand bookshop.

Your Guide to Positive Life

7. SLEEP AND REST

You will intuitively feel that you need time to regenerate in order to maintain full energy. This moment of „charging the batteries" takes place during your daily dose of sleep and rest.

The regeneration of our body is most effective between 21:00 and 1:00 at night. For this reason, it is extremely important to go to bed early so that you can get up in the morning full of energy for the whole day. You also need to prepare yourself properly to sleep – that's why I encourage you so much to practice the Evening Ritual, which calms your thoughts and relaxes your body.

Try not to stay in bed too long in the morning – it is likely to make you feel lazy.

Remember!
What you eat for dinner matters. Choose easily digestible food. This could be something warm, like vegetable cream soup. The last meal should be eaten about 2 hours before bedtime.

<u>Exercise:</u>
1. Enter the time of day and the idea for dinner into your daily schedule. Write down what time you will go to bed.
2. Plan your daily rest halfway through the day – it could be a moment to read, a short nap or a quiet walk. It is important to not only enjoy life, but also gather energy for your next experiences.
3. Look at your daily plans. Do you make sure to change your activities and body position in them, e.g. do you work in the garden/workshop (movement), then read a book (sitting), cook dinner (standing position)? This is important for your body, but also for maintaining a balance of energy. Performing the same tasks for a long time may cause unnecessary fatigue. Make your days more varied!

Your Guide to Positive Life

8. ASSERTIVENESS

You may be wondering how assertiveness is connected with positive energy. I will show you a few situations comparing an assertive and an unassertive person helping others:

Unassertive person	Assertive person
Lets others take advantage of their kindness.	Sets boundaries to help those who really need it.
Puts the needs of others first.	Remembers to take care of themselves, too.
Solves difficult issues for others – weakens and makes the person in need dependent on themselves.	Knows it's all about smart help. Gives the rod, not the fish. Strengthens and supports.
Builds their life around the affairs of others and thus takes over their stress.	Separates other people's affairs from their own. Maintains balance in life.

How do you feel reading the left side of the table above? Stressed? Tired? Overburdened with responsibility for the lives of other people? Do you feel like you are losing energy?

Remember!
The beauty of life lies in caring for others. It affects your inner development. However, **an assertive attitude will help you keep your life energy for yourself** and avoid the people who want to manipulate you.

I write here about wise help, because this is what I usually talk about with people who come to me for lectures and write letters to me. I think **you want to help** like they do, but sometimes you feel overwhelmed by the excess of things and taken advantage of by others.

What does "assertive" mean?
„*Capable of expressing his/her needs, feelings and opinions openly and unambiguously.*"
Dictionary of the Polish language, PWN

In order to become an assertive person you need to know your needs, feelings and opinions, so I am glad that you are working with this Guide. Step by step, you will discover what is important to you. Self-confidence and self-love will give you the courage to openly express who you are. **It is never too late for this!**

I'm sure the people around you will be surprised when you start changing. However, think that ultimately, it will be beneficial both for you and for your family and friends. **This will help you to heal your relationships and make yourself fully known**.

Exercise
1. Now think about what you have spent too little time on in your life. Maybe you didn't have enough time for physical activity? Or maybe for spiritual and intellectual development? Write everything down on a piece of paper. Consider it honestly and without any excuses. Why didn't you become more involved in these things?

2. Now write down something you've devoted too much time to. Maybe to help other people who didn't need it at all? Maybe to do things you didn't want to do, but didn't know how to decline? Maybe to fulfill not your own desires, but those imposed by the environment? Write everything down on a piece of paper and reconsider why you did so.

I hope that the above exercises have made you aware of the importance of taking care of your needs and feelings, and thus an assertive attitude. **Use your life wisely! Do not waste energy!**

Workbook 2

Your Guide to Positive Life

9. HEALTHY EATING AND EXERCISING

Your body is a versatile machine that needs good fuel to produce vital energy. Therefore, take care of proper nutrition and exercise.

Start taking care of yourself and eating healthy food right now. Don't wait until you get sick! Listen to your body.

This one simple activity – **planning your meals** – will help you not only to change your eating habits to healthier ones, but also save time and money.

Instead of eating the same monotonous meals every day, buy instant soups or take away food because you forgot to defreeze something, just a few minutes of planning once a week. **Even if you live alone, it's worth taking care of yourself by preparing home-made meals.** Or perhaps make an appointment with a friend or loved one to cook for each other every other day? This will strengthen your bond!

Here are some tips to help you plan weekly:

1. **Use seasonal ingredients**
   Avoid the problem of planning a meal for which you will not find any ingredients in the store.

2. **Maintain variety**
   This will give you the pleasure of eating and the right nutrients for your body.

3. **Choose quick and easy recipes**
   If you haven't been fond of preparing meals so far, make it easier for yourself by choosing simple and quick recipes. Write down the tastiest recipes so you can go back to them.

4. **Create a meal template**
   Create a schedule of at least five meals per day. It is best to eat meals with 3-4 hour breaks inbetween to avoid harmful fluctuations of sugar in your body. Plan your cooking time as well.

5. Make a shopping list
   It will save you time during shopping and help avoid putting unnecessary products and snacks in your basket. You will also save money.

Take care of your nutrition – would you serve fast food to a small child? No!

If you have a problem with cooking during the day or plan to spend the day away from home, try preparing 5 boxes of food the previous evening.

Remember!
Even the best diet needs support in the form of exercise. Healthy eating and physical activity are an integral part of our lives.
Ideally, you should spend half an hour at least three times a week on moderate exercise. After 6 weeks your energy level will increase by 20-30%! That is why I still encourage you to do our morning and evening stretching exercises. Thanks to them, the level of endorphins, i.e. the hormone of happiness, increases.

<u>**Exercises**</u>
1. From now on, during the evening summaries in the calendar, answer two additional questions:
   - How much did I exercise today?
   - What did I eat today?

   Be honest with yourself. In this way you will be able to track your actual progress in taking care of your health and happy life.

2. Make a motivational list.
   Record all the benefits you gain by changing your eating habits and increasing your daily physical activity.

Workbook 2

Your Guide to Positive Life

10. ANGER AND JEALOUSY

I would like to talk to you about some emotions that can drain your energy if you experience them often and unchecked. Did you know that emotions can be practiced? Start to develop your emotional intelligence so that your emotions don't control you anymore.

Anger

Where does anger come from? Make a list of the things that have made you angry and upset lately, and write next to them what the root cause of your anger was.

For example:

Situation	My feelings
Another customer cut into the cue in front of me.	I felt ignored and overlooked.
I helped someone financially when they asked me to, but it turned out that they spent the money on something completely different.	I felt cheated and lied to.

Anger can manifest itself externally by screaming, unpleasant words to another person or aggressive posture. When supperessed in your heart, it makes you feel as if something is lurking beneath the surface and wants to burst out at any time. It is unbearable!

Don't waste your energy on anger. Therefore:
- Continuously practice assertiveness!
- Don't ruminate on annoying situations. Don't feed your anger.
- Always find the root cause. Ask yourself: „Why do I feel this way?".
- Change your anger into something positive! Let it be the impulse to change!

Jealousy

Once again please make a list of things/people you are jealous of. Think about the root cause of this feeling.

For example:

Situation	My feelings
„Others..." have more money than I do.	I am embarrassed that I can not buy what I want and when I want to, but have to plan every expense meticulously.
My friend is always seeing someone, she has a lot of friends.	I'm not interesting enough to make new friends at my age. I feel lonely and unwanted.

Jealousy very often results from low self-esteem. It's defined as „a feeling of annoyance caused by the lack of something that you really want to have and that another person already has".

Don't waste your time on jealousy. Therefore:
- Always consider your feelings.
- Love yourself the way you are.
- Start building your self-confidence

If you need it, go back to the exercises in the first volume of the Guide: „Remember – be yourself!" and „Self-esteem". They will show you the way to deal with the jealousy you feel.

Instead of saying: „I can't do it," say the words: „I can handle any situation because I trust myself". **Start turning your emotions into a positive force to act!**

Workbook 2

Your Guide to Positive Life

11. TOXIC PEOPLE

The emotions we talked about before are often a reaction to the people you surround yourself with. Avoid toxic people. How do you recognize them?

Toxic people are those who need you mainly to complain, to burden you with their problems and tragic stories. They flood you with their fears and negative opinions about other people. Do not be someone's garbage can! You are not a dirt filter.

Exercises
1. Create a list of people you are in contact with. Write down the answers to the following questions for each of them:
   - What makes me happy about this relationship?
   - Am I as important to this person as they are to me?
   - Can I count on their support?
   - Do they enrich my life? Or maybe they drag me down?
   - Do I spend time with them out of habit or because I want to?

2. Mark which people give you energy and have a positive attitude towards life, and which are "energy vampires".

3. Arrange a meeting with people who, according to your list, support you and offer you an energy boost.

4. Think about yourself, too. Are you a friend to others? Have you become such a toxic companion to any of your friends, even though you don't want to? If so, think about how you can change this. An honest conversation is always a good idea!

Your Guide to Positive Life

12. SELF CARE

Together we reached the last exercise in the second volume of Your Guide to Positive Life. If you have also worked with Volume One, you have two months of intensive work behind you. **You will surely feel the influence of new habits on your life! Be sure to write to me about it!** I welcome every story I get. It's an inspiration and encouragement to continue my work.

Now find time for healthy rest – take care of yourself!

When you are exhausted, you often get irritated and have trouble concentrating. Fatigue can have a lasting impact on your mental and physical health. Long-lasting rest deprivation weakens our body's immunity, and as a result we are more likely to become ill.

That is why it is so important to relax after a tiring day.

Before you proceed to enhance your life with volume III of the Guide, do a few pleasant things for yourself. Working on the Guide, although beneficial in its effects, is also a great effort on your part. Reward yourself!

For example, I will celebrate finishing to write this Guide this way:
- I will cook a healthy and delicious meal for myself – I will decorate the table with porcelain tableware and fresh flowers. I want to feel that this is a special occasion,
- I will take a long, warm bath with relaxing music – to relax my body after all the time spending time at the keyboard,
- I'm going to sit down with my favorite book in my chair and I won't have to do anything more.

Now you go and do something for yourself, too!

Sincerely,
Kasia Dorosz

Your Guide to Positive Life

MOTIVATIONAL SENTENCES FOR YOU

"Your time is limited, so don't waste it living someone else's life.
Don't be trapped by dogma – which is living with the results of other people's thinking.
Don't let the noise of other's opinions drown out your own inner voice.
And most important,
have the courage to follow your heart and intuition.
They somehow already know what you truly want to become.
Everything else is secondary."

Steve Jobs

"A journey of a thousand miles begins with a single step."

Confucius

"Emotions were like wild horses and it required wisdom to be able to control them."

Paulo Coelho

"Twenty years from now you will be more disappointed by the things that you didn't do than by the ones you did do. So throw off the bowlines. Sail away from the safe harbor. Catch the trade winds in your sails. Explore. Dream. Discover."

Mark Twain

"The only person you are destined to become is the person you decide to be."

Ralph Waldo Emerson

Your Guide to Positive Life